BETHANN GREENAWALT

Infertility Minefield

This book was professionally typeset on Reedsy.
Find out more at reedsy.com

Whenever you find yourself dobting if you can go on, just remember how far you've come. Remember everything you have face, all the battles you have won and all the fears you have overcome. Then raise you head high and forge ahead, knowing You Got This!

Contents

Preface

If you are reading this, likely you or someone you care about is in the middle of the infertility minefield. As I sit on my back deck writing this many years after my battle, the trauma, scars, and wounds of this part of my life are still with me. I get teary even now as I think about all I went through. I want to write and share parts of my story in an effort to help you deal with your struggle right now. I think this may be the first time I've ever been truly transparent about this struggle. When you are deep in the trenches, you feel like you are alone and don't have a sense of any end. I want you to know that you are not alone.

Hi, my name is Bethann and I have dealt with infertility most of my child-bearing years. Infertility is something that happened to me but it doesn't define me. I now have two beautiful children that fill my every day with joy and amazement. These two people who are growing up so fast came from me (and my husband of course). I can still hardly believe it.

So what exactly is infertility? It is defined as the inability to get pregnant after one year of unprotected sex. Notice it doesn't say "actively trying to conceive". From that I gather any couple with routine sexual intercourse should get pregnant even by happenstance within that one year. The CDC says that approximately 1 in 5 women or 19% will fall into that category. With that many women and men struggling to get pregnant, why is it still such a taboo topic? I think it is really personal and often we don't let people see that side of ourselves. Remember, Instagram, Facebook, Snapchat, and TikTok are really only highlight reels of our lives and we aren't often showing the time it took to prepare for that highlight and the reality of the everyday life.

Let's face it, infertility sucks! It can lead to depression and anxiety. It has the ability to drain your finances and put a strain on your marriage. If you have any of these struggles, that is normal. I implore you to seek some guidance and support from a professional or at least some friends. You need an outlet to keep sane.

I hope that as you hear the minefield I traversed, you will be able to find a path to keep you protected from the mines. By sharing my story, I hope more women will be empowered to talk about theirs. I want you to come out of the battle unscathed or at least with minor wounds and no mines will blow you apart!

The Infertility Minefield

**My battle to become a mother
and avoid being blown up in the process**

1

The Age of Innocence

I remember back when I was planning to get married, I went to the OB-GYN for an annual exam and to ask about getting birth control. I wasn't ready to have children. I remember telling her that I only have periods every 3 months. I asked her if I should be concerned about that when I do decide I want to start a family. She said the only concern was that it may take longer if I only cycle every 3 months. Red flag #1!

It's funny to think back now without those rose-colored glasses on. I see the start of that very dangerous path but I didn't know it, then. In my ignorant mind, there is no minefield. Why in the world would this doctor say that? You see, I am a nurse and rather well educated, but even I didn't know the world of infertility. But a board-certified OB-GYN should or at least I thought they should.

So I went on my merry way, marrying my best friend and establishing our lives together. We wanted to wait for a few years before expanding our family. I decided to go to school for my master's degree in nursing and a family would just make things more challenging.

Fast forward another two years and we have now been married almost four years. I just finished grad school and was taking a month off between school and my new job. This was the first time I ever had a few weeks where I wasn't working. It was amazing. My husband, Rob, took me on a surprise trip. He planned our travel destination in the mountains of North Carolina in January. We hiked through the woods in newly fallen snow. It was wonderful. I remember having a conversation about stopping birth control and letting whatever happens, happen. It was freeing and I was ready to take that next step. I wasn't sure where this path would lead but I had decided that perhaps it was time to think about having a family.

I was starry-eyed and dreaming of baby things: names, nursery, having a pregnant round belly. You know those dreams, right? It hadn't been shattered into a million pieces yet. I went into this new phase of life with a mindset that I knew it may take a little longer. Oh well, I still have time on my side. At this point, I am only 27, almost 28. Often people would ask if we were planning to start a family and I pretty much tried to be nonchalant about it and give vague answers because I didn't want everyone asking me all the time as I knew it may take a while.

Hindsight is 20/20, they say, and my ability to look back and see what that younger woman was going to go through is telling. I wish I could warn her. I see all the explosions that scar her today and I wish someone had told her how to navigate through without the same hurt. This is truly the age of innocence. I didn't know what I didn't know. Well, those rose-colored glasses I mentioned earlier? They were about to be ripped off and crushed underfoot.

Mine avoidance tip #1: Understand that any journey where you are emotionally vulnerable to the ups and downs there might be along the way, can lead you to expectations that may not be met right away. If those expectations aren't fulfilled, it could prove to be a bomb that will blow up in your face. Give yourself time to understand the process and grace for your emotions that will bubble up to the surface. Find a way to make some peaceful time for you and your spouse. Don't allow the process of having a family become an obsession.

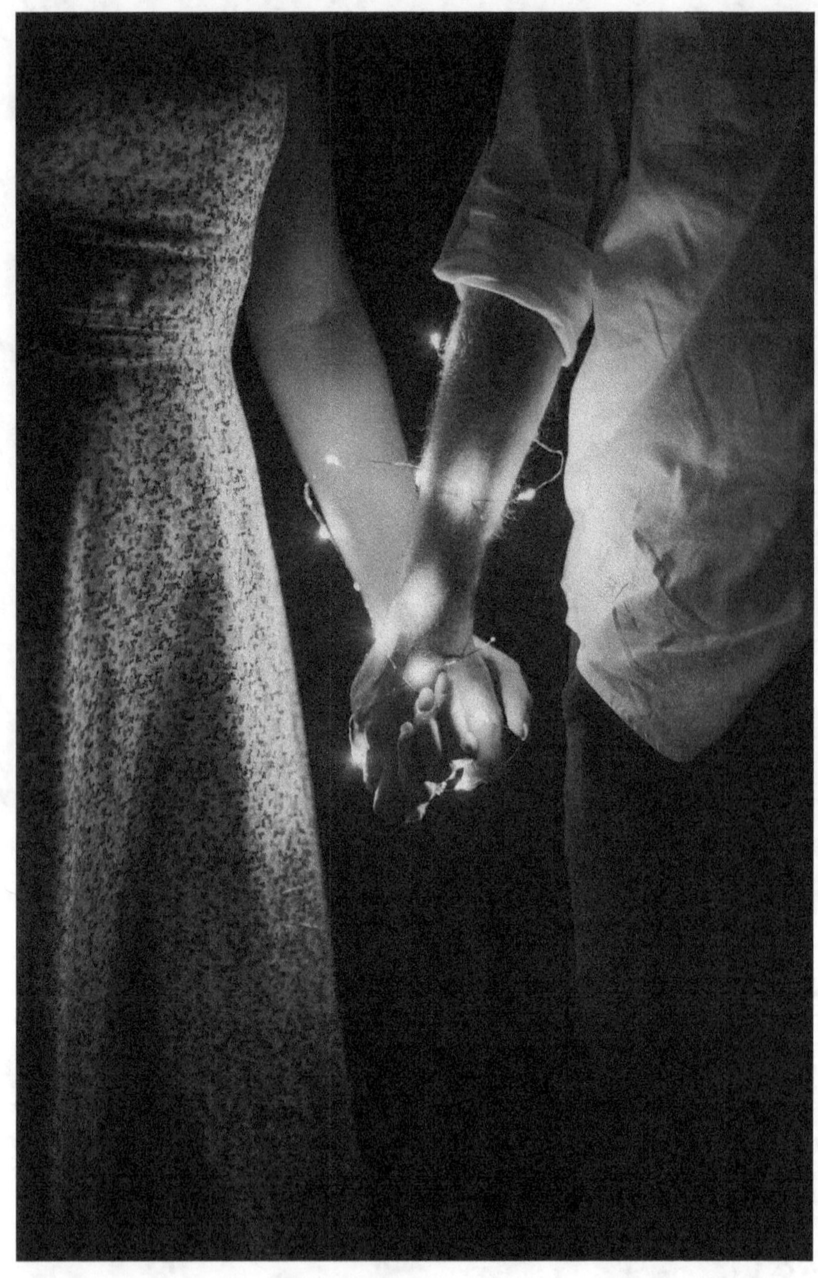

2

Why Is This So Hard?

After more than a year of trying, I started to think I need to know more about fertility. I mean, an educated woman should educate herself about something she doesn't really know much about. I learned all about the hormones in the cycle and fertility charting. All of this started a descent into many hours spent searching online for answers and obsessively monitoring my fertility chart. I started taking herbal supplements and after months of charting, I realized that I wasn't ovulating. I even had a family member tell me that maybe God just didn't want me to have children. Ouch. That hurt. Not ovulating should have been my Red flag #2, but I was stubborn and didn't want to elicit outside help so I continued on my journey alone. That minefield was just over the next hill.

After more research, I decided to try natural progesterone cream which I applied to my forearm daily and after 3 months of using the cream, I actually ovulated and of course I knew this because I was charting my temperature every morning before I even moved a muscle outside of bed. A few weeks later, I was away with my husband and didn't pay close attention and of course, my naivety kicked in and I stupidly didn't realize why my period did not start because remember, I hadn't had normal cycles off birth control since my late teens. Eh hem, it turns out I was pregnant! I was so excited. I was about 7 weeks along. I called the Dr. and made my first appointment. Around 8 weeks, we told our families we were expecting. That was a bit premature. At 9 weeks, I had a miscarriage. That bomb was a major hit to my feelings and it took me a while to recover. So I did what I do best: hide and research.

I self diagnosed myself as having PCOS (Polycystic Ovarian Syndrome). It should have been something my OB-GYN had picked up on and counseled me about years before. I mean, I was obese, had hair growing where it didn't belong, had irregular cycles and after tracking my temperature and cycles, did not routinely ovulate either. After that miscarriage, we decided to seek medical help from my local OB-GYN. Not the first one who told me it may just take longer to conceive but another one in the same practice whose wife I knew personally. He basically told me I was getting old and that we needed to hurry up. In order to explain things to my husband, he tried an analogy using cars. He said that when I was younger my eggs were more like a Ferrari but as I age, the quality of the remaining eggs are decreasing and that it was like a Pinto! Can you believe it? I mean, how dare he? Really? I was so mad at that. He agreed that I likely did have PCOS but didn't really bother to address it. He provided me with Clomid and sent me on my way.

So that was the beginning of the medical journey I would undertake during my many years trying to conceive. Little did I know what lay ahead.

Mine avoidance tip #2: Take the time to educate yourself on fertility and how to conceive. I mean, real, medical science and not hokey stuff. I started wrongly by being stubborn and not seeking medical assistance sooner. I researched supplements which weren't wrong but also not all that helpful because my issues were bigger than the minor abnormalities those supplements could help. When you are educated, you know what to expect. I think I may have known more about fertility than my local OB-GYN at that point. No offense to them but a lot of them do not specialize in infertility so they only do the very basics. An educated person is no longer naive and less like to step on the mine of ignorance.

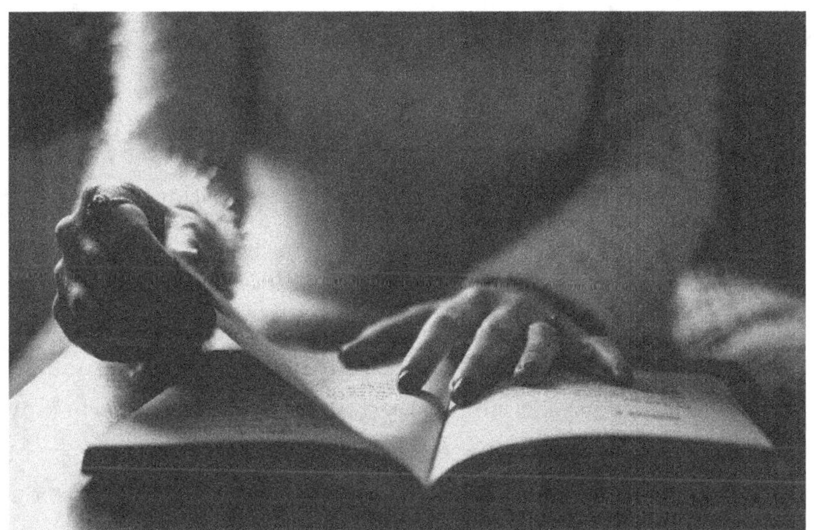

3

What The Heck Is Wrong?

Now, I am sure I have PCOS. I tried Clomid and the first time: Bam! I am pregnant again. Wow, that was fast. This must have been what I needed. I was cautiously excited. I mean, I got pregnant before but had a miscarriage. This time, since I had a history of pregnancy loss and I am under the Dr.'s supervision with medication, the office sent me right away for a blood test for beta hCG (Human Chorionic Gonadotropin), the hormone produced when pregnant. I was definitely pregnant but the levels weren't rising as they should. Oh boy. Here we go again. After a week or so of monitoring, they brought me in for an ultrasound which did not show any intrauterine embryo. Um, what? Dr. says I likely had a miscarriage and the levels would go down. Nope, they kept rising slowly. Now they don't know what to think. The day they wanted me to come in for another ultrasound, my car wouldn't start and my husband was away working. I had to get AAA to come and jump my car and likely my battery would need to be replaced. While I waited for AAA, I just broke down and sobbed. At the office the Dr. said I likely have an ectopic pregnancy and that we needed to do surgery right away before it became life threatening. Really? I mean, wasn't there enough drama already?

So two days later, on a Saturday morning, I found myself at the hospital for the "emergency" procedure because the Dr. said it couldn't wait until next week. And sure enough I had an ectopic pregnancy.

To add insult to injury, the whole next week had been a planned vacation. We were going up to the family cabin with my husband's entire family. The hospital wanted to keep me for observation but I refused and said we had to keep to our schedule. We went home that evening and finished packing and drove the 4.5 hours up to the cabin in the dark. I rested for a few days there and the family was especially accommodating. I didn't do any cooking or cleaning. I sat on the swing and read for hours. Then after that short bit of recovery, we drove home.

OMG! I forgot that the carbon dioxide that they pump into your body to inflate the abdomen has to come out eventually and the entire drive home, I had such terrible pain everywhere in my central body that every bump in the road was pure agony and I was in tears. Rob didn't know how to help me. I was emotionally and physically broken. The next day we flew to Fort Lauderdale, FL for a brief getaway. It was supposed to be a happy time together but instead I felt so empty.

Infertility has many causes. The strictest term is for those who can never get pregnant, either there are no sperm or eggs being ovulated or there are abnormalities in the organs of either the male or female that cannot be fixed. The other term I've learned about is subfertile, meaning the possibility of conception is still on the table but there are medical reasons that make these couples' dreams of having a family so much more challenging. Most people with infertility struggles will fall into this category. Things like low sperm count or motility, infrequent ovulation, poor egg maturation, endometriosis, imbalances of various types of hormones, polyps and blockages in the fallopian tubes. PCOS is a subfertile condition and affects 6-12% of women in the US. Many of them are unaware and remain undiagnosed.

Mine avoidance tip #3: Again, education here is another key. Understanding the ins and outs of infertility. Knowledge is power! But my tip here is to seek appropriate medical help. I didn't realize my regular OB-GYN was not equipped to diagnose and treat my issues. Surround yourself with the right level of medical professional for what you are trying to achieve. I took it "low tech" for way too long. My journey now is over 3 years. You can avoid the mine of time wasted by knowing when to get advanced help.

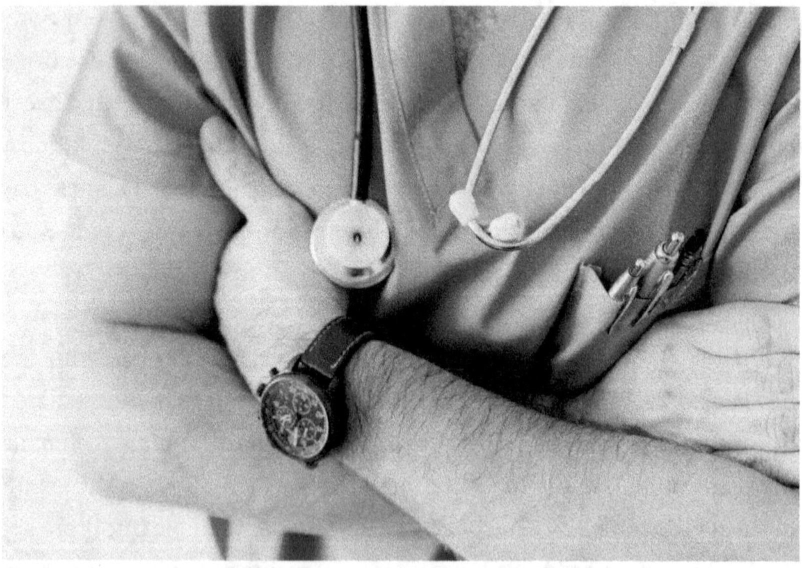

4

The Friend Zone

Another thing I found difficult to deal with during this whole process of trying to conceive is how lonely it feels. My husband was so supportive and while infertility was happening to "us," it really is on a whole different level for me and I think women in general. Society has conditioned us to want to be mothers from an early age. Weren't you mommy to your baby doll? I know I was.

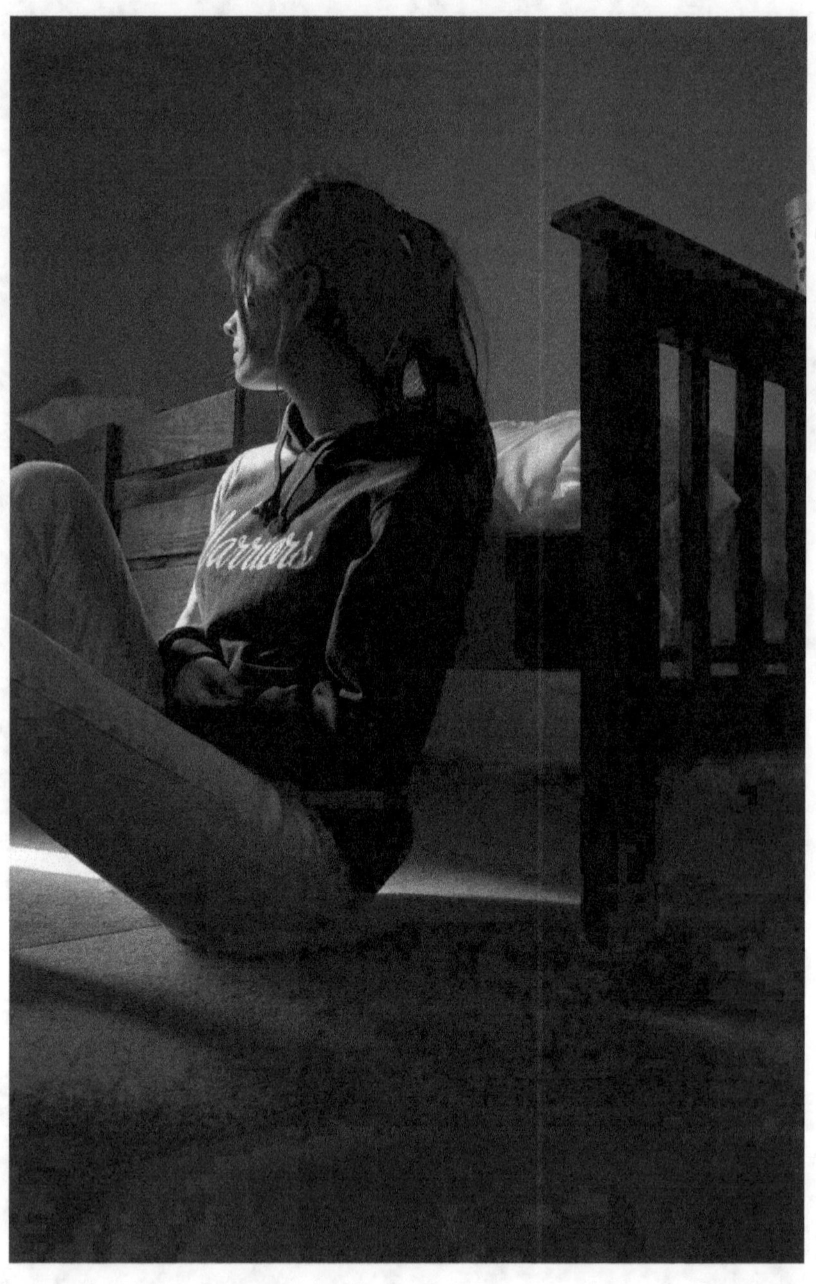

It really is part of nature to want to procreate. It is how we as a species continue to thrive on the earth, right? So not being able to make that very basic function happen left me feeling like a failure. Because sex in general is a private thing, trying to make a baby is also something I kept mostly to myself. My family knew we were having difficult becoming parents and that we were seeking medical intervention, but I didn't share everything with them.

Because of this level of privacy, well-meaning friends and family didn't really understand what I was going through and would often make comments about, "when are you going to have a baby?" and "I hear you had a miscarriage. I am so sorry but maybe that was for the best and you'll be pregnant again soon." I know they didn't have the whole story because if they did, they wouldn't have said those things, but how can I really share what is going on? It is simply so very personal. Something that I really only talk about with my husband and some online chat groups that I joined.

The part that hurts the most is when I see friends and family getting pregnant all the time around me. I mean, logically, that makes sense that cousins and friends will get pregnant because we are all around the same age, mid 20's to early 30's. That's the time to have a family. But getting invited and attending baby showers was a two-edged sword. I was genuinely happy for these loved ones, especially the ones that I knew also struggled to get pregnant. But on the other side of that sword, it cut deep to have my arms empty and no party for me.

Each event I went to got harder and harder over the years. Step carefully now, there are mines with hair triggers everywhere. The potential of getting hurt is high in this extremely fragile emotional state.

Mine avoidance tip #4: Go easy on yourself. You know where your limits are emotionally. Share what you want and keep private what you want. Don't let friends suck the life out of you. If you can't stand to attend another baby shower, then don't go. Send a gift and your love but guard your heart. I struggled with that because I am a people pleaser so I took part in every event and then it got me depressed for a week or so afterward. Learn from my mistakes and set boundaries.

5

Getting Out The Big Guns

After the ectopic pregnancy, I still was too stubborn to waive the white flag of surrender. I kept at the Clomid for another 5 cycles. No, I did not get pregnant again but I was ovulating so at least that part worked. My husband's cousin went to a fertility specialist and had success so I thought perhaps I should up my game. I scheduled myself with this specialist and now we are on a whole new level of things.

My first appointment and impression of this man was that he was so kind and genuine. I really thought working with him would be a good thing for me. The first hurdle though is all the testing! Because of my history there was an ultrasound, lab tests and even more. If you are starting on this journey, prepare to throw modesty out the window. Everyone needs to see your nether regions on a routine and regular basis.

What they don't warn you about is that some of these tests are emotionally fraught as well as physically daunting. I had a sonohysterogram where they push saline into the uterus and then observe with ultrasound looking for fibroids or other structural anomalies along the cervix and walls of the uterus. That wasn't too bad and was performed in the doctor's office.

Next on the checklist was the HSG (hysterosalpingogram). This is a radiology procedure with fluoroscopy where they observe in real time the injection of dye into the uterus and track where it flows. Now this procedure was rather cumbersome with having a speculum attached and a tube running dye. The Dr. at my foot end, the radiologist managing the imaging, and the radiology technician who, God bless her, grabbed my hand as tears spilled down my face. This procedure was extremely painful for me. They made me turn side to side to observe if the dye spills freely from the fallopian tubes. For me the right side was blocked and the Dr. was trying to put some force with the dye and that was causing all the pain. That was the side where I had the ectopic, so the tube was spared, however it was now damaged and I would not be able to conceive with any egg released from the ovary on that side.

Sigh. I feel like I've now had a triple whammy. First off, I don't ovulate regularly on my own. Secondly I have had pregnancy loss which often happens in women who are subfertile. And thirdly, I now have even less chance of getting pregnant because typically only one ovary will release an egg each month and now one tube is blocked so on those months where the right ovary releases the egg it is another month further from my dream of motherhood.

Even my husband was tested with his special sample. He passed with flying colors! In fact his count was off the charts at almost a billion sperm in one shot. So now it was time to come up with a plan. For me, the doctor recommended we start with medications and monitored cycles to confirm ovulation and time intercourse. There are many courses of treatment that can be prescribed depending on the cause of infertility anywhere from oral medications like Clomid to injectable hormones, IUI (Intrauterine Insemination), IVF (in vitro fertilization), or surgery (pelvic laparoscopy). This was likely one of the cheaper pathways but still a drain on our finances.

Mine avoidance tip #5: Be prepared that testing can be a few months, especially if you require some surgical procedures like a pelvic laparoscopy. I know you have already been trying for a while and every month waiting feels like you are getting further from your goal. But remember, that getting to the root issues of your infertility is time well spent and you will come out of this with a solid plan which likely will save time in the long run. Patience. That is the key here.

The tests themselves can be rather uncomfortable. What helps you through pain? Do you meditate or pray? Take some time before these tests and procedures to find the calm in the middle of that storm.

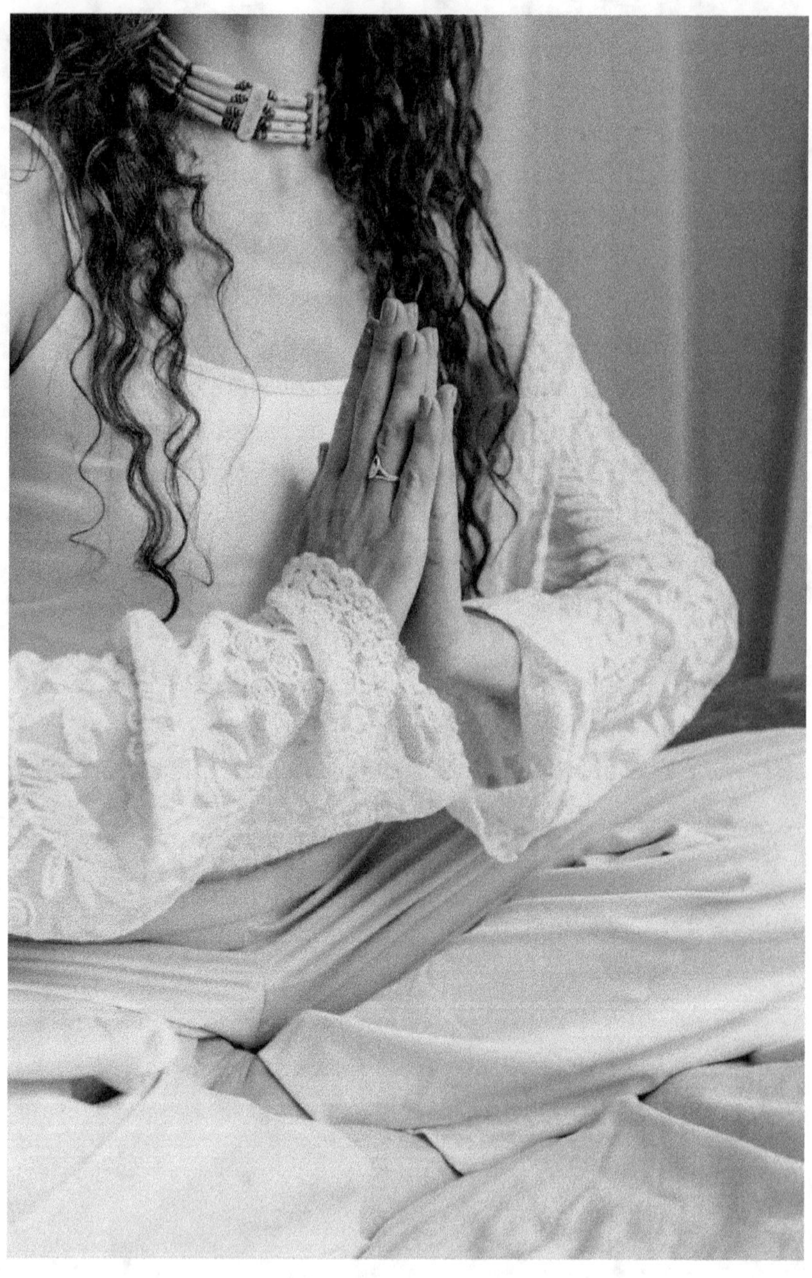

6

Treading Down The Treatment Road

There are many ways to treat infertility based on the causes. Since I definitely had PCOS, was able to get pregnant previously and now have a blocked tube, the best choice of treatment was hormone injections aimed at stimulating the ovaries to produce several eggs so that hopefully we can get an egg to release on the left side every cycle. The specialty pharmacy sent the medications by overnight mail and I opened a large box of a lot of needles and vials. It was rather intimidating. I began this new path by calling the Dr. office when my cycle began and getting an ultrasound on day 3 (yes, even while bleeding). Then I started injecting myself every day. Remember, I am a nurse and I've given loads of shots to people, but I had never given one to myself before. I remember pausing and looking down at my abdomen and taking a big breath before that first injection. Mind you, I was sitting at my desk at work doing this because I had to give myself the injection at the same time every day which happened to be while I was still at work.

This starts the routine of several days of injections, then going to the

Dr. office first thing in the morning for bloodwork and ultrasound, followed by a phone call from the clinic nurse in the afternoon telling me what dose to inject myself that day and when to come back in the office for the next lab and ultrasound. I usually had to go 3 or 4 times before they said, "Ok, go ahead and take the hCG injection tonight." You read that right. The medication used to induce ovulation is the same hormone produced when you are pregnant. This one is not as easy as the abdomen injections. This one goes in a large muscle: your bottom. I was concerned about giving this one to myself as it was also a large needle. I instructed my husband how to give it to me. Of course, that's not all I had to do. I had to have intercourse that night and the next two nights. It can prove challenging to be "in the mood" when everything else about this process is all clinical.

Then they brought me back to the Dr. office for another ultrasound to confirm that I did indeed ovulate. All these office visits also put a strain on my work. I had to share with my boss what was going on because I needed to be late to work many mornings because of the labs and ultrasounds. She was very supportive and allowed me to flex my time to account for that. It was a little stressful to then work late on those days.

Let's face it, everything about this whole process is stressful. The endless appointments, the financial challenges, the hormones wreaking havoc on your body and emotions, the shifting of work, the waiting. There's a reason they call it the Two Week Wait. That is the time between ovulation and menstruation and it is fraught with the emotional ups and downs magnified by the increase of progesterone: breast tenderness, bloating, fatigue, depression, and anxiety. During all this time, I had to continue with inserting a specially formulated vaginal suppository of progesterone twice daily. That was a creamy mess. During this time, it is easy to have high hopes and then burst into tears within minutes of each other. It's like being on an emotional rollercoaster that you have little control over.

For me, this treatment process had to be repeated 3 times until I was pregnant again. But only for a week. My hCG levels were not rising fast enough and my progesterone was dropping. This is now my third pregnancy loss. I was really starting to feel like this was never going to happen. I started this journey at the end of age 27 and now I was 32. Was I ever going to achieve the dream of being a mother?

Mine avoidance tip #6: If you are going through treatments, find a buddy. I did get to know a few women at the Dr. office but we didn't always get there at the same time so it was hit or miss. My doctor did offer a support group and while I wasn't able to attend due to my work schedule and the office being a bit of a drive for me, I would highly recommend connecting with other people who are going through this process at the same time as you. There are online groups, too. I found support online to be valuable.

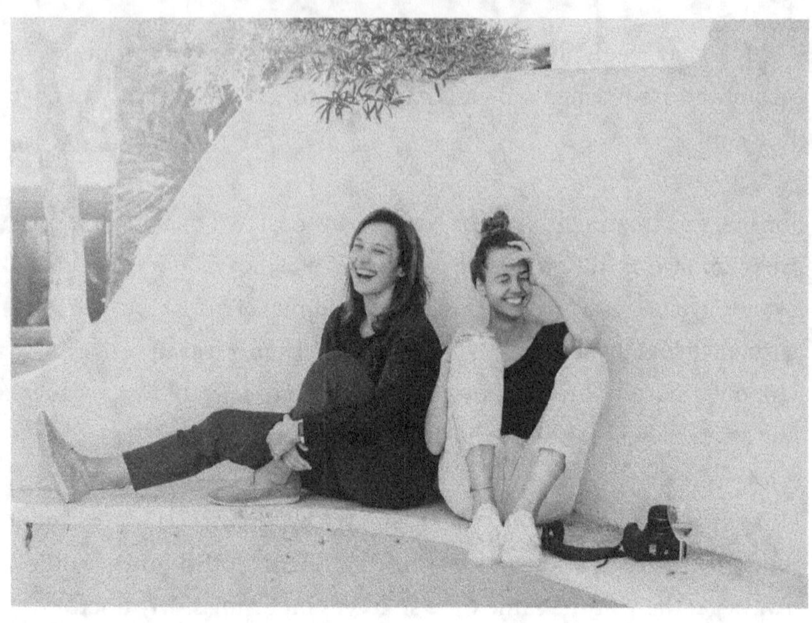

7

Cautiously Optimistic

I have now been seeing the fertility specialist for 7 months. I have completed 3 rounds of injections and added another miscarriage to my tally. The Dr. could see that the injections were having the desired effect and after resting for one cycle after the miscarriage, we started the 4th round of injections and timed intercourse. For some reason, I remember being optimistic about this cycle. So it was nearly the end of my Two Week Wait and I was in Nashville for work (rarely do I get to travel at work so this was an unusual circumstance to begin with). So in true drama fashion, I was due for my testing to see if I was pregnant during the middle of my trip. I had to find a hospital lab that would allow my Dr. to fax an order for the lab tests to be performed. Then I had to sneak out of the conference and get a cab to take me to the lab and of course a cab ride back. And of course, the hospital was like 12 miles away so $50 later, I was back in the conference. Then in the middle of my lunch break, I get a call from the nurse at the Dr. office. I was pregnant and my numbers actually looked good. Could this really be The One!?!

I wanted to be guarded but I also couldn't help but be elated as well. I didn't want to tell my husband over the phone. I wanted to wait and tell him in person. It was going to be a long 3 days because even though I found out on Wednesday and I was flying home on Friday, my husband was going to be away for work and I wouldn't even see him until late on Saturday. At the hotel gift shop, I found this cute baby size yellow t-shirt with a teddy bear "cowboy" on it and it said Nashville. I decided I would give this to my husband as a gift and have it be my way of telling him that we were expecting. It was a bittersweet moment. I had high hopes but it was hard to truly be excited.

This is where a whole new level of anxiety sets in. In my mind, other pregnancies ended because the eggs weren't all that good and the embryos likely had genetic abnormalities not compatible with life. It's not easy putting that worry aside. In the fertility specialist's office, they follow up with labs and ultrasounds until 6-8 weeks of pregnancy. I can't tell you what a joy it was to see my little baby's heartbeat at 6 weeks. I had never seen this in previous pregnancies. But there is still that feeling of walking on eggshells (or perhaps not wanting to step on a landmine again). I don't even think we told our families for a few weeks and the general public did not know we were expecting until after that first trimester mark.

You see, the battle scars of the past linger throughout the entire pregnancy. I tried not to worry too much, but it is very hard. A lot of women who fall pregnant easily and don't experience a loss, don't really understand. That's okay, it's not their fault. I just held on to that cautious optimism for the journey.

I know nothing goes normal for me. Even my birth story has some level of drama with it. I forgot to mention that my first job in nursing was as a labor and delivery nurse. I know what can and does go wrong in labor and I had thought many times over the years preceding my pregnancy that when it comes time to deliver, everything that can go wrong, will go wrong for me. Murphy's law, right? Well, not everything went wrong, but I did have some challenges in the weeks preceding the birth and some trauma at the time of delivery, but I will spare you the details as this is not the point of my book. Infertility leaves that indelible mark on you even in the midst of the joy that you are supposed to have when having a baby.

It was late in the day that my precious Emma was born by c-section. She was my medical miracle. After nearly 5.5 years from when I decided to stop birth control, I finally had the baby who made me a mother. Life was forever changed. I remember the tears that rolled down my face as they held her next to my head while still in the OR. I couldn't even reach out and touch her because the spinal medication was so high up on my body that my arms were numb and I couldn't move them. They took her to the nursery to be weighed and bathed while the PACU kept me for quite a long time. It seemed forever for the medication to wear off enough for me to move those arms. Two hours later they took me to the women and babies floor. As they wheeled me down the hall, I heard a baby cry and instinctively, I knew it was my little girl. She was hungry. I could finally put this infertility path behind me.

Mine avoidance tip #7: If you do achieve pregnancy, marvel at every moment of it. I had a hard time putting aside the feelings of the past losses and it affected how I felt about my pregnancy for a long time. Don't let your fears and anxiety rob you of the joy that comes with being pregnant.

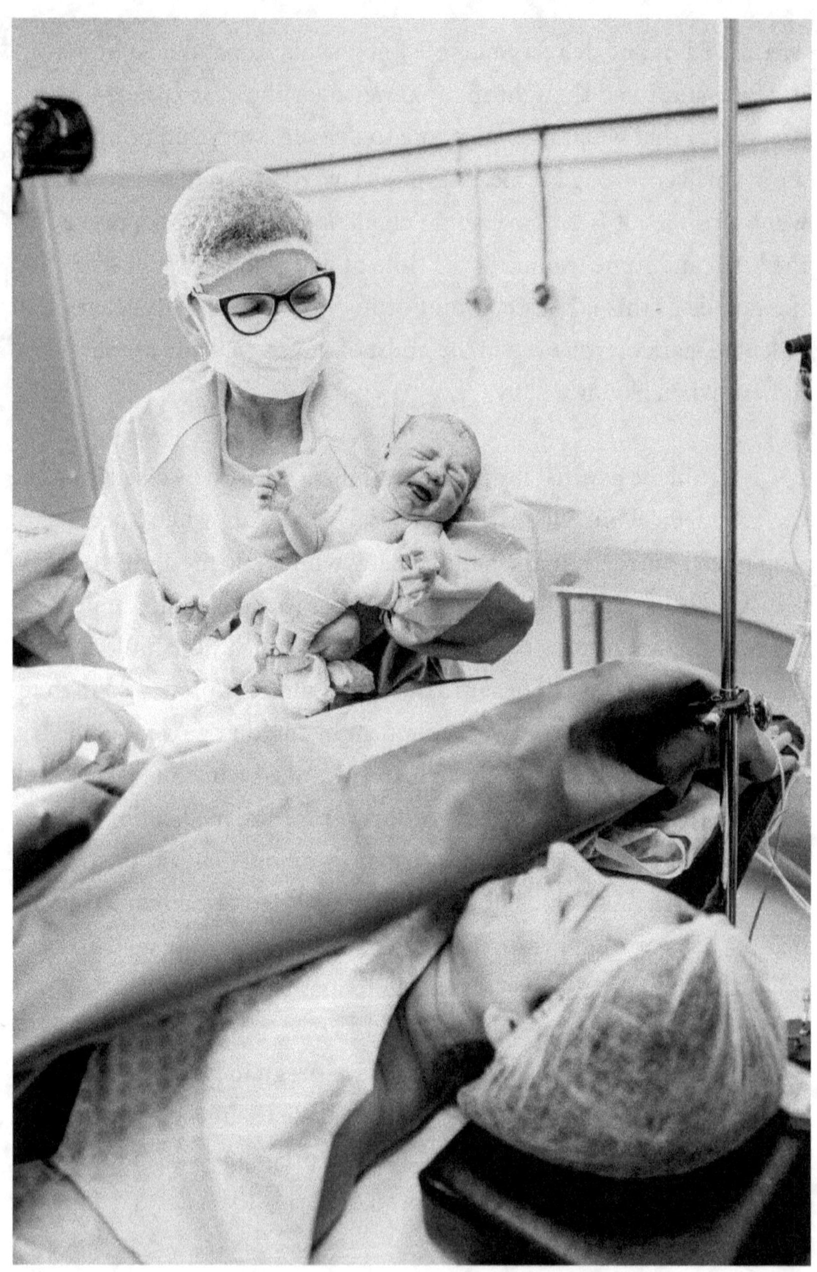

8

Is It Possible?

I put so much energy in being a mom to my little girl, but I knew in my heart that my family was not complete. Around the time she was 18 months old, I talked to my husband about starting the process of trying to conceive again. Despite my diagnosis of PCOS, ever since delivering, I had regular monthly cycles. I wasn't doing the temperature charting so I couldn't be sure that I was ovulating but at least it seemed to be an improvement.

I started back to charting and following my cycle more closely and made an appointment to go back to the fertility specialist. I wasn't going to mess around anymore. I was mentally and emotionally prepared for this journey through the minefield again. I had my consultation and then I was scheduled to go back for discussion of the plan when I had a positive pregnancy test. I called the specialist and they followed up with bloodwork and ultrasound. I could hardly believe that I had only been back to charting for 3 months and really only "trying" for one month. Could it really be?

This time God smiled on me and blessed me with our second child, Caleb. He was a different kind of miracle to me. I remember keeping it a secret from my husband for a little over a week. Just long enough for me to get a t-shirt that said "Big Sister in Training." I know, another t-shirt, but I couldn't resist the irony in that. I put it on her one evening and called my husband up to the nursery to help me. It took a beat for it to sink in for him. I allowed myself to be excited. I just knew this time, it was going to work out. I had Caleb when I was 35. Being a "geriatric" mother adds a whole other level of complexity to pregnancy and his birth story was also a bit of drama, but in the end he was a healthy, happy, large baby at 22.5" long and 10 lb. 14.5 oz.

Mine avoidance tip #8: Grace. You have to give yourself grace and allow yourself to feel all sorts of emotions. I really liked being pregnant. I had built walls around my heart though and spent a lot of time feeling guilty about being happy to be pregnant again so easily this time. Just sit with those feelings for a moment and be real with yourself.

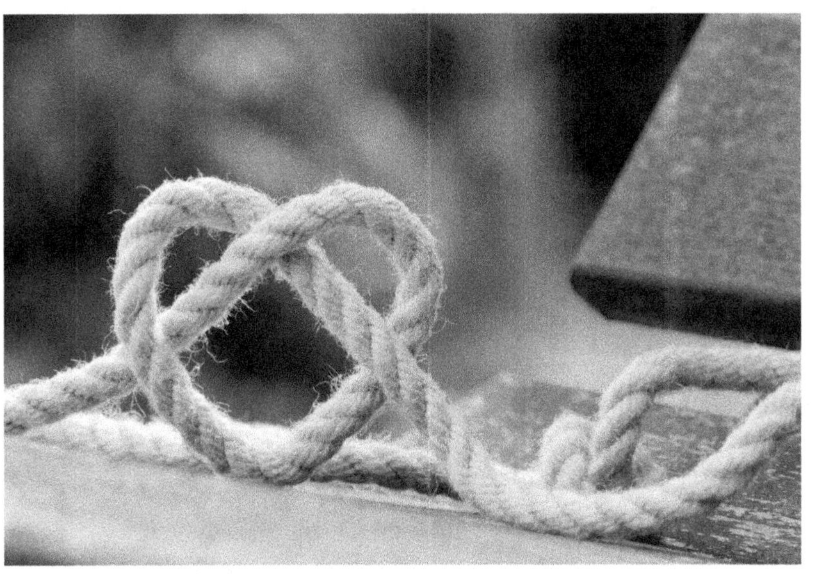

9

When Time Is Not On My Side

You would think that at age 37, I am happy and content in my life with two small children. In my heart though, I had always dreamed of having four children. I was not quite ready to give that up. We now live in another state and I decided to try low tech again and give myself 6 months to try for another baby. I asked my new OB-GYN for Clomid and I started charting. In the first month of taking Clomid, I was pregnant again!

I could hardly believe my luck, but I should have known better. In my case, this again was not a viable embryo and I had my 4th pregnancy loss. It helped that another woman at my church also had a miscarriage at the same time as me. I felt like I could talk to her a little bit about it. I had a church family that was really supportive. I sang in the choir and when I told the group at rehearsal that I was having a miscarriage, they prayed for me and I truly felt that love and support.

Sigh, it just didn't seem to be going my way. I took a full 6 months of Clomid and never got pregnant again. That friend at church got pregnant again pretty quickly and ended up having 5 more children over the years for a total of 7 and another woman at church had 2 more children in the time I was trying to conceive my third. Ugh.

I thought that was going to be the end of my journey, but I wasn't quite ready to give up. I looked online and found a highly rated reproductive endocrinologist in my town and reached out to him for assistance. He did require some testing but we were able to get my records from my prior specialist so he didn't make me do everything again. He needed to see if my egg reserve was good and if my husband's sperm was good. Since I was even older now we wanted to maximize the shocking low chance of conceiving. I vaguely remember him saying we had a 10% chance each cycle. This time the recommendation was for injections followed by IUI (Intrauterine Insemination).

I want to mention that before seeing the fertility specialist, I decided to really take charge of my health. I joined a medically monitored weight loss clinic. I followed a strict high protein diet with their protein supplements and went twice a week for weigh-ins. It was a pretty intense program and I lost 40 pounds in 6 months. I felt good and was proud of my accomplishments.

I went into this with my whole being and started going to acupuncture with a wonderful woman who specialized in infertility. Her name even gave me a sense of rightness with the world, Faith. I saw her twice a week for many months. It felt awkward at first but she really made me feel good and I was glad I added this complementary treatment to my medical path.

I didn't mention too much about the cost of treatments in this book up until now. It is a real issue for many couples. I am so glad to hear that some states have been requiring health insurance companies to provide some level of coverage for infertility treatments. In my case, however, I had no such coverage. I even worked for the federal government but it was not part of my insurance. Everything was going to be out of pocket and I had to sign financial paperwork with the specialist. They gave me a baseline price per cycle. I don't remember now exactly what it was but somewhere around $2000 per cycle. Finances have always been a struggle for us. It is something we argue about frequently. I had some savings but definitely not enough for too much of this. This was going to be a challenge for us but we were ready to give it our all.

The injections were much like before but the IUI added a whole different spin on things. No longer did we have sex to make a baby. It made everything so clinical. Romance was nowhere to be found. As expected, my husband's sperm were off the charts. The hormones gave me several "target" eggs each but I still only had one working fallopian tube, so that reduces the chances. The first IUI cycle, I got pregnant! Wow, I remember thinking this was amazing.

I should have known, a new kind of drama was to ensue. My hCG levels were rising slowly. A lot of times in early pregnancy, they look to see that the numbers double every 2-3 days and it was doing that but just barely. The Dr. was not hopeful and neither was I but it still seemed to be hanging in there. The numbers weren't high enough to be able to see an embryo on ultrasound (typically you can see that by the time the level is 2000) but they tried anyway. No sac found. In the middle of all of this, we had a trip planned to go visit my family over 900 miles from where we lived. We had to go and I was in the middle of this drama.

This pregnancy would not clearly go one way or the other. My Dr. called me while I was away and said that he was worried that it could be another ectopic and that I should go to be seen right away. My husband took me to the Women and Babies hospital in town. It was a freestanding hospital only for women. I was seen in their "emergency" triage area. We were there for four hours for labs and ultrasound. I had to go back for two more lab tests in the week we were in town. Again, the levels continued to rise but no pregnancy was found anywhere. Eventually the hCG levels started to drop and a week later I had my miscarriage. This drama lasted from the first positive pregnancy test until 9 weeks. That's over a month of uncertainty! Craziness!

Mine avoidance tip #9: Rely on your partner. Sometimes, you can't help but step on a mine no matter what you do. I had no control of the situation around me, but no matter what, my husband was there for me. He shared in every cycle and loss. I know that he might not have felt the same level of loss, but he is my best friend and was my shoulder to cry on.

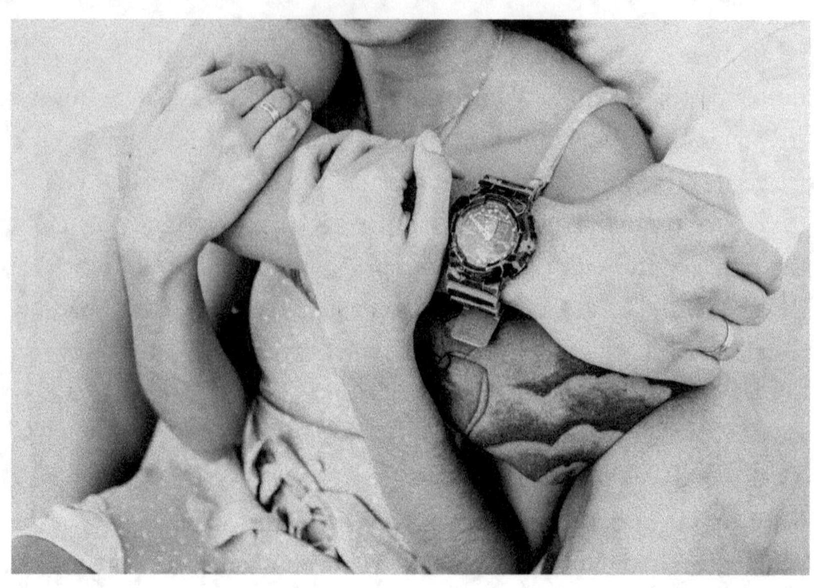

10

When Enough Is Enough

I had now gone through loss #5 and this one seemed to be even more drama than any other one. It took several months to pick up the pieces after that one. The Dr. even insisted that I take a few months off before attempting another IUI. Once I was emotionally and physically on an even keel, we began again. I had no time to waste, I was 40 years old now.

In the middle of all this, a new level of stress ensued. We had decided to move back to our home state though not exactly near where we grew up. There were a lot of decisions to be made but nonetheless, there was work to be done on the fertility front. So I trudged on through the battlefield. I think part of me was a little emotionally vacant and stunted with each passing month. At the very moment of our move, I had literally completed my third IUI and we moved during that Two Week Wait. I had even promised to notify my acupuncturist, Faith, of the outcome of that last cycle. Unfortunately it was a bust. Not only did I not have a baby after that year, I now had some bit of debt as we had spent around $14K for these medical treatments.

35

Now I was in a new town with no friends or family nearby and I felt like this path had come to an end. Rob had other ideas. His love for children had blossomed over the years and his desire to have another one had not waned. He wanted us to keep trying. We lived in a very rural part of the state and there was no specialist nearby. I made a deal with my husband that I would find a local OB-GYN and just try low tech again and that this was our last chance. This Dr. was extremely kind and gentle, I really loved her. She happily gave me Clomid again. I knew my chances were slim, but I felt I would give this one more shot.

We did another 6 months of Clomid but never again got pregnant even though I knew I ovulated each time. Over the course of 8.5 years of trying to conceive, I got very good at knowing how my body felt with ovulation, temperature tracking, effects of hormone shifts, etc. I had also peed on so many ovulation strips and pregnancy tests that I could see lines in my sleep. I was now 41 and even though I didn't want to give up, I had that frank talk with my husband. We just knew that we couldn't keep going. This whole process had really taken its toll on both of us. My heart still wanted to be a mother again but my head won out this time. It was hard. Really hard.

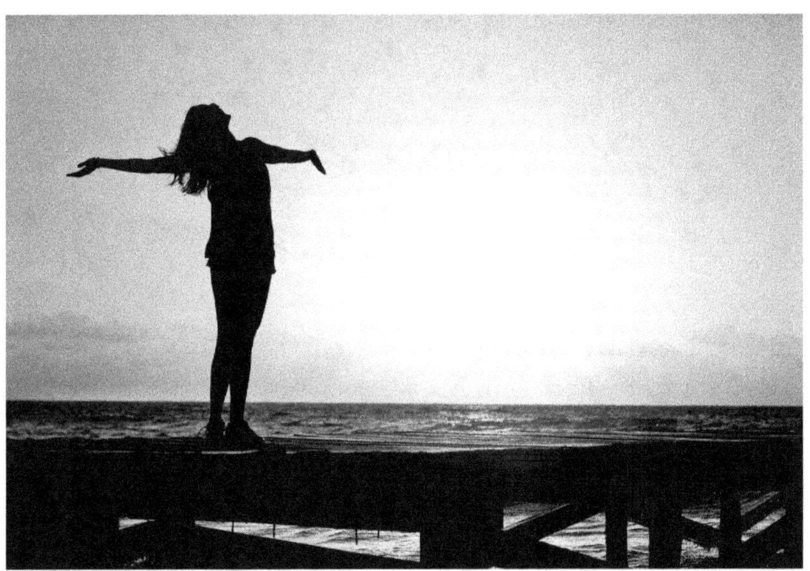

Mine avoidance tip #10: Release that unmet expectation. It is not easy but when you know it in your core, you can let go and find that lightness inside. I can say that I held onto some bitterness for a really long time. I wasn't a happy person for quite some time. I hope you can find a way to be free regardless of if you have a baby or not. There is so much to be found in life; just living and breathing day in and day out. Watching the sunset and knowing there is a tomorrow.

Epilogue

This is my story. Each of us has our own, very personal story on the path to motherhood. Some of you are just starting on this path that leads through a field of mines set to explode if you veer one way or the other. You may find your way out with relatively little scars. Some of you will continue to struggle for years to come and feel like there are constant explosions that throw shrapnel everywhere and you may emerge battered, bruised, and scarred . And some of you may have to leave the minefield of infertility to follow a different path. Whatever your outcome, I hope that you find peace and comfort and that your strength as a woman becomes the cornerstone to throttle you forward through life.

I can sit here years after my battle has ended and finally put pen to paper and share what I went through. I have a strong faith and truly believe there was a reason I went through all this. God has never left me alone in this struggle. I still have moments when I wonder what could have been, but I know that at this moment, I have peace. My life is full. It may not have been exactly the life I had hoped and dreamed for but it is a fulfilling life. My children are everything to me. They are precious and sent from God to me. I can only hope that the woman I became because of the struggle is better because of it. I am strong. I am filled with compassion. I have battle scars but I am still pushing on.

I hope that my words have been practical and provided you with some comfort, helping you know that you are not alone in the minefield. Many have gone before, others are right there along with you and whenever you need help, don't hesitate to waive a white flag and get help from your spouse, a friend, counselors, and medical professionals. You are loved and you are not defined by this struggle.

If you have found my book to be helpful to you, please leave a kind review on Amazon.

Citations

American Pregnancy Association. (n.d.). *What is HCG?* Retrieved July 17, 2022, from https://americanpregnancy.org/getting-pregnant/hcg-levels/

Centers for Disease Control and Prevention. (2020, March 24). *PCOS (Polycystic Ovary Syndrome) and Diabetes.* Retrieved July 17, 2022, from https://www.cdc.gov/diabetes/basics/pcos.html#:~:text=PCOS%20is%20one%20of%20the,beyond%20the%20%20child%2d%20Bearing%20%20years.

Centers for Disease Control and Prevention. (2022, March 1). *Infertility FAQs.* Retrieved July 17, 2022, from https://www.cdc.gov/reproductivehealth/infertility/index.htm#:~:text=In%20the%20United%20States%2C%20among,to%20term%20(impaired%20fecundity)

Content source: Division of Reproductive Health, National Center for Chronic Disease Prevention and Health Promotion

Jabeen Begum, J. B. (2021, October 1). *Seeing a Doctor for Infertility: Questions and Treatments.* WebMD. Retrieved July 17, 2022, from https://www.webmd.com/infertility-and-reproduction/guide/understanding-infertility-treatment

Mayo Clinic. (n.d.-a). *Female Infertility.* Retrieved July 17, 2022, from https://www.mayoclinic.org/diseases-conditions/female-infertility/symptoms-causes/syc-20354308

Mayo Clinic. (n.d.-b). *Infertility.* Retrieved July 17, 2022, from https://www.mayoclinic.org/diseases-conditions/infertility/diagnos

is-treatment/drc-20354322

Pugle, M. P. (2022, January 28). *Symptoms of High Progesterone.* Verywell Health. Retrieved July 17, 2022, from https://www.veryw ellhealth.com/high-progesterone-symptoms-5185751

SingleCare Team. (2022, February 15). *Infertility statistics 2022: How many couples are affected by infertility?* The Checkup by SingleCare. Retrieved July 17, 2022, from https://www.singlecare.com/blog/news/ infertility-statistics/

The Cleveland Clinic. (2020, December 13). *Infertility Causes.* Retrieved July 17, 2022, from https://my.clevelandclinic.org/health/ diseases/16083-infertility-causes